Allergies, Asthma and Computer Use:

The Contributory Effects of Computer Use to Allergies and Asthma Trends

By
Adetutu Ijose

Published By

Jointheirs Publishing

JP

Allergies, Asthma and Computer
Use:
The Contributory Effects of
Computer Use to Allergies and
Asthma Trends

Jointheirs Publishing
Jointheirs Activities Incorporated
www.jointheirspublishing.com

ISBN –1-46116-181-9

EAN –978-1-46116-181-3
Printed in the United States of America

Allergies, Asthma and Computer Use:

The Contributory Effects of Computer Use to Allergies and Asthma Trends

An Important Caution

The advice given in *Allergies, Asthma and the Computer User* is based on my personal experience when in 2006 I became the casualty of the effect of long term computer use on my health.

Like everyone else I did not realize that computer use had an effect on health and so I did not take the sneezing and headaches and so on as a warning that something was going on that needed a few changes in the way I handled my computer use.

I had to learn to accept the fact that computer use hurts as a consequence of suffering life-threatening consequences of long-term computer use the doctors could neither understand, diagnose or treat.

What I am sharing in this short book are things I wish someone had told me many years ago, which would have spared me so much suffering

I was forced to go to the human computer user manual we call the Bible where with prayer and consistent study, I began to understand the human code of existence, its violations inherent in computer use and the various measures put in place by our maker before hand with which we need to comply in order to minimize the effects of these violations and avoid devastating consequences.

These understandings are documented in my various books available at amazon.com and other store. A complete listing is provided at the end of this book. I will advise you to get copies of then to increase your understanding of the issues we will be discussing in this book.

This book is informational and is a guide that contains both advice and instructions. It is essential that you read the entire book carefully and that any decision you make be discussed with your physician before proceeding.

This books seeks to help computer users and those around them identify when computer use is the reason for allergy or asthma like symptoms they or their loved ones may be manifesting and as well as provide advise on how to avoid reaching that stage.

It also provides suggestions on how to manage and reverse the situation. Please note that the result will vary with each individual based on a vast array of issues including a person's perseverance and persistence in carrying out suggested practical lifestyle changes and other advises provided.

This book is not meant to replace the advice or service of a health care provider who knows you personally. An essential element of taking responsibility for your life and health is getting regular checkups and working in partnership with medical professionals

If you are under treatment for any computer-related behavioral disorder or if you suspect you might need such care, you must discuss any insight you gain from this book with your doctor before starting.

Table of Contents

Chapter 1
Asthma Statistics

The Centers for Disease Control and Prevention (CDC) statistics for asthma for 2009 [1-1] is as follows

1) Number of noninstitutionalized adults who had asthma: 17.5 million

2) Percent of noninstitutionalized adults who had asthma: 7.7%

3) Number of children who had asthma: 7.1 million

4) Percent of children who had asthma: 9.6%

For 2006 [1-2] the figures were

1) 9.9 million U.S. children under 18 years of age (14%) had ever been diagnosed with asthma; 6.8 million children (9%) still had asthma.

2) Children with a parent who had more than a high school diploma were more likely to have respiratory allergies, hay fever, and other allergies than children with parents who had less education

3) Nine percent of U.S. children under 18 years of age suffered from hay fever in the past 12 months, 12% from respiratory allergies and 13% from other allergies

4) In 2006, there were 9.6 million children in the United States (13%) who had a health problem for which prescription medication had been taken regularly for at least 3 months

For 2003 – 2005 [1-3]

1) An estimated 7.7% of people (22.2 million) had asthma

2) Rates decreased with age; 8.9% of children (6.5 million) had asthma compared to 7.2% of adults (15.7 million).

For 1980 to 1998 [1-4]

Asthma period prevalence among children 0–17 years of age more than doubled, from 3.6% in 1980 to 7.5% at the peak of the trend in 1995.

Chapter 2
What is Asthma and what are allergies

According to the World Health Organization (WHO) [2-1] "Asthma attacks all age groups but often starts in childhood. It is a disease characterized by recurrent attacks of breathlessness and wheezing, which vary in severity and frequency from person to person. In an individual, they may occur from hour to hour and day to day

This condition is due to inflammation of the air passages in the lungs and affects the sensitivity of the nerve endings in the airways so they become easily irritated. In an attack, the lining of the passages swell causing the airways to narrow and reducing the flow of air in and out of the lungs."

While allergies are defined by the Mayo Clinic [2-2] as follows:

"Allergies occur when your immune system reacts to a foreign substance such as pollen, bee venom or pet dander.

Your immune system produces substances known as antibodies. Some of these antibodies protect you from unwanted invaders that could make you sick or cause an infection.

When you have allergies, your immune system makes antibodies that identify your particular allergen as something harmful, even though it isn't. When you come into contact with the allergen, your immune system's reaction inflames your skin, sinuses, airways or digestive system.

The severity of allergies varies from person to person and can range from minor irritation to anaphylaxis — a potentially life-threatening emergency. While allergies can't be cured, a number of treatments can help relieve your allergy symptoms."

The advanced data for vital and Health Statistics for the CDC – Number 381 published in December 12 2006 revised December 29, 2006 - The State of Childhood Asthma, United States, 1980–2005 by Lara J. Akinbami, M.D., Office of Analysis and Epidemiology[2-3] says the following about asthma

"Millions of children in the United States are affected by asthma, a chronic respiratory disease characterized by attacks of difficulty breathing. An asthma attack is a distressing and potentially life-threatening experience.

Scientific advances have greatly improved the understanding of the mechanisms that cause asthma attacks and have led to effective medical interventions to prevent morbidity and improve quality of life. Yet, the burden in prevalence, health care use, and mortality remains high. Asthma remains a significant public health problem in the United States "

Chapter 3
Artificial Light and Light Sensitivity

Sometimes people find themselves having light sensitivity i.e. unable to look comfortably at for example the screens of their cell phone. Further they find this happening when they come up with symptoms that resemble allergies or asthma.

This can be especially troubling for people who are adults with no history of asthma or allergies but who are always on their cell phones, computers or who sleep with artificial light on in their rooms all night or work in artificially lit rooms for long hours.

The constant bombardment of artificial toxic light probably affects the production of melatonin at night for those with light on all night in addition to the exposure of nerves and their receptors to toxic artificial light and toxic chemicals present in the artificial light fields.

For those on cell phone, or exposed to various artificial reading lights such as fluorescent, incandescent and so on and maybe TVs, the constant bombardment of their nerve receptors by toxic artificial light all day gradually compromises the receptors creating infection. In all these cases there is potential for compromise of the immune system.

Immune system compromise can occur because what maintains our bodies are light fields or electromagnetic field generated in the body by a complex system that breaks down the light fields we receive from natural sources – the sun moon and stars into that which can operate in bodies like ours and all others that operate on earth e.g. animals and plants to produce the activities we need to operate as terrestrial bodies connected to the earth from which we are made.

Medical science tells us the cells in our bodies do not talk directly to each other and actually are controlled and manipulated by messaging network of biochemicals called neurotransmitters.

For anyone who has never heard about biochemicals, these are light fields that act chemically hence the name biochemicals. They can neither be seen nor touched as light cannot be seen or touched but we feel their effects. They power, run and maintain our physical bodies.

In fact our behavior and activity as humans depend on the balance of these biochemicals in us.

Examples of biochemicals include such things as neurotransmitters (Serotonin, Gamma Amino Butyric Acid – GABA and so on), hormones (estrogen, progesterone and so on) and enzyme (bromelain, papain and so on)

The user manual we call the Bible puts it starkly. It tells us the physical flesh on its own has no life and depends on a second realm the soul realm where decisions and choices are made and behavior and activity is determined. It tells us the soul receives life that it uses in operating the body.

Hence both the manual and medical science tell us that, our body cells do not communicate directly with each other it is the biochemicals that pass messages to them through the nerve network. Nutrients are passed to them through the blood under the instructions of biochemicals. Hence the physical we can see is given life and maintained by an unseen realm where the biochemicals reside. This is the soul realm.

The soul realm is given life and powered by the spirit realm as the manual tells us. This life is given by and under the direct control of our maker alone. It is used to start and terminate the process of our existence here on earth.

Everything in creation has life. It is coded in all things by our maker and provides us with the ability to move around, make independent choice and operate here in creation.

Without life we cannot operate and anything that is lifeless is toxic to the soul area, which needs an abundance of life to operate the physical. When we expose ourselves to lifeless light and chemicals we are exposing the soul to something it cannot work with. It is like introducing a virus into a computer system. It uses up the resources and begins to compromise the system. That is what artificial life does in us.

Indeed light sensitivity is a phenomenon that usually arises as a result of the overexposure of the nerve receptors and sensors to artificial lifeless light without a counterbalance of exposure to sunlight to reduce the effect of the toxicity introduced by artificial light.

Artificial light is not of the same composition as sunlight it can never be. For, light cannot be seen or touched it is its effect we see and measure not light itself. In addition, sunlight contains life i.e. the spirit of life from our maker, which recharges us with life every time we are in sunlight or are exposed to its rays directly or indirectly via a medium such as glass.

This life stimulates our brains to produce inhibitory neurotransmitters such as GABA that calm us down and prevent excitative ones such as noraldrenaline from over firing with excitement in the presence of light and its high-powered energy enabling, us to operate comfortably on the earth.

Sunlight permeates all natural elements hence some go through the wall of buildings but the quantity is not enough to handle a room for example totally lighted with fluorescent or other artificial lighting all day.

One thing I suffered and noticed in others was that in many cases, in normal allergies you could have a running nose. When it is artificial light the nose does not run but the nose is blocked and the nose and lungs congested. There could also be nerve pain, upper back and upper chest pain

Hence many people find themselves sneezing and exhibiting symptoms that resemble allergy and asthma in the office. When they get home they switch on all the lights all night and even sleep with the light on. In addition to this they watch television till late disturbing their body's ability to produce melatonin a biochemical that operates as hormone and a neurotransmitter as well as the most powerful antioxidant in the body that is responsible for repair and growth functions while we sleep.

Obviously melatonin deficiency is a very big problem and has been indicated in many studies as being a contributory factor in the onset of cancer and other debilitating diseases that arise from a compromise of the body's natural repair and maintenance system

Please get hold of my book *Lessons I Learned the Hard Way* if you would like information on detailed research work that has been done by my scientists all over the world on this issue. To make things simple for the purpose of this short book, I will cite the conclusion of only one set of scientists.

Anisimov VN; Zabezhinski MA; Muratov EI; Popovich IG; Arutiunian AV; Oparina TI; Prokopenko VM in their article on their research findings in the journal *Biofi zika* [Biofi zika][5-2] concluded that the data obtained indicated that the exposure to radiation from personal computer video terminals had a marked biological effect and may adversely affect the health of users due to its negative effect on nocturnal melatonin and other chemicals.

When I was suffering from life threatening consequence of computer use that exposde me to a high volume of artificial light with little sunlight exposure, I came up with something that resembled allergies and asthma too. Claritin did not work neither did any other conventional method of treatment.

As I learned the way the body was coded to be by studying the human machine user manual we call the Bible, I realized the function of the sun and the life coded in us through it.

I also came to an understanding of the effect of the falling of the water that used to be above the earth as rain in the account of what happened in the days of Noah.

I was able to understand the effect of that event and why humans were authorized to eat animal protein after that.

They needed more iron, amino acids and other nutrients that plants could not supply in sufficient quantity to handle the increased exposure to sunlight.

They also needed to handle the increased need for energy that the earth that had been cursed and was now difficult to cultivate required.

This gave me a clear understanding as to why we need to have sunlight in abundance in our system in the technology age. He made provision for them after the flood for that time and any other event that would require additional sunlight exposure.

This is just one a simple example of the many insights I received that enabled me come up with a treatment plan when medical science could not help.

Our maker had made provision for the increased need for energy to cultivate the hard ground that the sun was supplying to be a blessing and not harm us.

And so the sun stimulates our brains to produce additional inhibitory neurotransmitters and other biochemicals to keep us calm in spite of the high voltage of electricity we are exposed to in sunlight.

The same level of voltage of artificial light would completely burn us alive because there is nothing in it to provide protection. That can only be provided by our creator/programmer.

Part of the reason I became ill is that the various offices where I had worked over the years in the corporate world, were usually only lit by artificial light and many times with closed doors.

In cases where the doors were left open there was usually only one door and hence no cross ventilation.

This meant that the air was consequently imbalanced and polluted with artificial light with no sunlight to provide antioxidants and calming biochemicals to manage the imbalance and pollution in my body.

In addition to this, at that time I finally crashed health wise, I lived in an apartment that was located against the direction of the sunlight and so even though I had many windows, I did not have much sunlight and had to depend on artificial light for lighting and reading indoors all day.

In some offices where there were glass windows, because I did not realize I needed the sunlight, I treated it as something to be shaded against and would let the light in partially until it became too hot as a result of the glass and I would pull down the shade leaving me at the mercy of the artificial light.

Many at times I would sneeze or find the air stale or even have headaches and find it difficult to breath. I thought all that was temporary difficulty and never expected it to have lasting accumulative effect as I always felt better after I got home, had a short walk or none at all, ate and went to bed.

No one had told me that because all this was contrary to my natural coded way of life there would be a lasting effect.

Everything I read in the news seemed to suggest our bodies would adjust to the difficulties over time.

It said that as a result of evolution our bodies would evolve to handle anything we exposed it to.

Even though people talked about the human machine and use terms such as genetic code DNA code etc. apparently no one took into consideration the meaning and consequence of what it means to be coded.

It means there re limitations put in by the programmer of the code to make it come up with the end result called the human being and we can only operate within the flexibilities provided in the code. We will never adjust to anything not provided for us to adjust to.

The user manual we call the Bible tells us no changes will be made to the code until this whole system is wiped away and replaced with a new one which this current system is the raw material for.

When it reaches the point for the change, that is when all things will change into that which is perfect and all natural, nothing artificial will be there.

It will all be holy, no rebellion, sin etc will be there because only those who on this side have chosen to and have successfully learned to want only that which is good and holy and to choose that which is right automatically can and will upgrade to effortless perfection and glory.

That is the beauty and essence of the free that our maker has given to all His creation. No one can make a choice for anyone else. We all have a choice but we must all be ready to face the consequences of our choices. For face it we will and there will not be a chance for a redo because this side would be over.

Consequently anyone waiting for their body to be able to operate on lifeless elements is in for a shock.

We were made to operate with life. Anything that is lifeless will always be toxic to us and there is a limit to which our souls, which is the area that produces biochemicals and that runs, maintains and repairs the body and through which life is passed to the body by the spirit can cope with before it becomes overwhelmed by lifelessness.

This is when the body begins to breakdown rapidly. This happens after an extensive period of time of the soul giving warning signs with issues that resemble asthma, allergies and other respiratory issues, eye issues, nerve issues and so on.

It is when we continue to pump in more and more lifelessness that it gets to a point where there is too much lifelessness and repair becomes impossible and a person could have a heart attack or some other failure such as liver or kidney failure that leads to death.

This means we are all accidents waiting to happen and ignorance will not save anyone. Ignorance did not save or help me.

Some of the measures I use and which I recommend that everyone adapt can be found also handle other issues discussed in this book and so to avoid repetition, I have written once in chapters 4, 5. 6 and 7

One thing I will mention here, wear only natural fiber clothing - cotton, wool, linen and so on when using the computer. When I was ill I discovered that every time I wore synthetic cloth I felt the electromagnetic fields of artificial light and a lot of statics.

I did some research and was surprised to discover that highly toxic compounds can be found in synthetic fabric.

Finally, please get a hold of my book *Lessons I Learned the Hard Way* for more comprehensive information on the issue of artificial light and light sensitivity. You can also reach me by email using information provided at the end of this book under "Notes to the Reader"

Chapter 4
The effect of air imbalance

Outside air automatically rebalance itself. That is the way our creator has coded it.

This balance is the atmosphere humans are coded to live in. We were created to be outdoor people constantly replenishing our biochemicals by the activity of the life containing light rays function that stimulates the production of the various biochemicals in the balance coded for our optimal performance as humans.

That is why we feel comfortable outside and feel calm in sunlight as inhibitory neurotransmitters are produced that counterbalance the excitative one that would other over fire as a result of the high voltage energy of the sun.

Indoors this balance is violated especially in today's world where most offices, homes and schools are all closed office buildings in a mistaken belief that we need to keep away the very sunlight we need.

Granted, the less pigmentation a person has, the less their ability to receive and retain the optimal level of sunlight needed by the body resulting in a situation whereby taking in optimal sunlight could destroy the very physical body it is designed to protect.

Pigmentation is our coded defense mechanism that protects the body from sunlight damage and enables the body to absorb all the sunlight it needs for optimal function.

Absence of this protective element can lead to skin cancer and other issues in the presence of prolonged sunlight exposure. Many people exposing themselves to unlimited computer light and other artificial light fail to realize that there could also be more serious damage form exposure to artificial light.

This is why those tanning beds that use artificial light are so dangerous.

One way to improve the ability of less pigmented people to stay in the sun for an extensive period is by using sunscreen.

Sunscreen is chemical and probably adds its own stress to the system. It can also be overdone in which case sunlight is not absorbed effectively and the effect of the stay in the sun is negated.

Many people think that we absorb all the light that gets into our bodies through our eyes. The truth is that we absorb most of the light our bodies use through our skin. We also absorb some light through all the openings in our bodies such as the nose, mouth, anus and so on.

When indoors there is a level of violation of this delicate air balance our bodies can tolerate. When the imbalance reaches a level of toxicity it has no flexibility for we begin to exhibit symptoms of discomfort manifested as headaches, sneezing, some light sensitivity when the toxicity has a light element, itchiness in some people and so on.

This is the body's way of registering discomfort in order to get our attention so we can make changes. Many a times we mistaken this for real sicknesses and medicate

when all that needs to be done are changes that reduce the toxicity of the air. There are people with real allergies and asthma not related to computer use. In such cases their symptoms may be exacerbated by computer use.
We will consider two main imbalances in this book
Air Ionization Imbalance

1. Air Moisture Imbalance
2. Air Ionization Imbalance:

An article on Negative Ions and computers presented by T. Neil Davis at the Alaska Science Forum on September 25, 1981[4-1] reported mounting evidence that ion concentrations in the air affect how people feel. The article stated that there was evidence that trends toward using computerized equipment may create special health problems and suggested a reason for this trend: This is a summary of what the article said

"Outdoor air contains about a thousand positive and negative charges (ions) within each cubic centimeter. Cosmic rays coming into the earth from the sun and elsewhere break apart air molecules and thereby create much of the ionization that exists in the air.

Since more cosmic rays come in at the high latitudes, the high-latitude air normally has a higher proportion of ionized air molecules or molecular clusters. However, in cities and in confined spaces such as offices where computer are used, processes take place to reduce the number of ions.

One important process is attachment of charge-carrying molecular clusters to pollution particles in the air.

When that happens both the ions and the pollution particles tend to be swept out of the air by the electric field that exists naturally near the earth's surface."

The loss of ion concentration is thought to be harmful because high ion concentrations seem to make people feel better—although just why this is so, doesn't seem to be clearly understood. High ion concentrations also apparently inhibit bacterial growth and perhaps foster plant growth.

The good effects seem to be attributable to high concentrations of negative ions rather than positive ones. In general, the concentration of both types go together, except in small volumes of air (perhaps only a few feet across)".

Davis also said that medical scientific works has proved the following advantages of charged ions:

1. Improvement of psychological and physical conditions.

2. Increased resistivity to diseases.

3. Decreased amount of bacteria in the room

4. Cleansing of weighed micro particles from the air

5. Easing of the effect of static electricity.

He said "The electric field caused by the positive static charge that appears on a cathode ray tube (CRT) screen of a monitor in normal operation strips the nearby air of negative charges, thereby depleting the negative-ion concentration in the immediate vicinity. Apparently, when this or any other means (e.g., air conditioning) lowers the ion concentration in a room, workers complain of headaches, lethargy, dizziness, and nausea.

Under the influence of this electrostatic field, dust and charged particles accumulate on the face and hands, provoking allergies, skin dryness, withering, and sometimes various eczemas".

In my various discussions with computer users I have found other issues including rashes especially around the eyes that never go away, burning eyes and light sensitivity (an issue we discussed earlier in chapter 3, chest congestion and bronchitis, lung murmurs and so on.

In my case I had lung murmurs and chest congestion. I have provided some of the measures I took to handle this issue further in this chapter and in chapters 5, 6 and 7 of this short book. A more detailed discussion is provided in my 300 page book *Lessons I Learned the Hard Way*". At the end of this book under Notes to the Reader information is provided on how you can obtain your copy of this book in print or ebook version.

Please note that it is not only operating computers that produce positive ions thereby throwing off the delicate air balance in the room. All sources of artificial light do this including fluorescent, incandescent, spectrum light and so on.

It is a fallacy to think we can create the same light we get from the sun artificially. Some people have developed breast cancer while trying to handle Seasonal affective disorders (SAD) and depression with spectrum light.

Do not play around with artificial light. It is lifeless and cannot do for you what the sun does. Nobody knows the composition of sunlight. It is impossible to do so all our science does is guess at it.

To handle SAD and depression get out into the sun, go for long walks as long as you can, wake up with the sun, do not watch television or work on your computer in bed, go to bed early and in a darkened room and change your diet to organic thereby avoiding chemicals, pesticides and herbicides and so on

For more on how to handle SAD and depression please get a hold of my various books including *Lessons I Learned the Hard Way*

Air Moisture imbalance
Just like air ionization. Outside air automatically rebalances itself. However indoor air especially with closed doors and windows, air artificially controlled by heaters and air conditioners is highly imbalance moisture wise.

In fact we need outside air to have water, which is why we feel uncomfortable in dry places such as deserts. The PH of outside air water is however different from that of tap water and so though washing the face often is helpful, it does not fully solve the problem.

Many people will also attest to feeling thirsty a lot during computer use.

In my case I was always thirsty and hungry and I also felt the heat of the air emanating from the computer screen.

If you are like me humidifiers and vaporizers do not work but only increase the discomfort.

Heaters and air conditioners dry up the air and in addition artificial light dries up the air because of the heat it produces.

As we have read, most of the light we take in is through our skin, the nerve receptors need moisture for this process. In addition our skin needs a certain level of water to be youthful and healthy.

When the air moisture is imbalanced all these processes are at risk. Because the computer screen generates light, this artificial light dries up the air around it and consequently the air around the face may feel dry and sometimes hot. One may also be able to feel the heat in the chest area or any other part of the body that is expose.

My advise is always be covered when working on the computer to reduce the amount of skin that has direct body contact with the toxic light emanating from the computer. Too much direct contact may prove too much for the body's stress management system to handle over time and could lead to devastating health consequences that could be misdiagnosed as more commonly known ailments with dire consequences.

The drying of the air around the face is what leads to the dry eyes syndrome that many computer users have.

That is why eye drops do not work because it is not the lack of the ability to create tears but the drying of the skin, making it difficult for eye nerves to receive and/or relay the messages required for tear formation. It could also result in infection of eye nerve receptors and other receptor issues.

The eye muscles and nerves like every other part of the body need moisture to operate well.

To handle this issue it is important to crack open the window to enable the air continually rebalance itself as close to outside air as it can indoors naturally. As I said humidifiers and vaporizers many not work. It did not work for me.

A second thing to do is to wash the face every night after cessation of computer use and moisturize the skin.

In addition there is special PH balanced water – face mist for relieving dry skin produced by a company called Biologic Aqua that one can spray regularly on the face while working on the computer.

This helped me a great deal. This coupled with cracking open my windows to let outside air in were some of the measures I took.

All you need to do is spray it on your face regularly. You do not need eye drops or anything producing tears as that is not the problem. It is a skin problem not an eye problem.

The skin nerve receptors just need a little help. That is the reason why trying to solve this problem with eye drops does not work. I did that too and it did not work for me too. So do not make that mistake. Just take care of the skin and the eyes will be okay.

Drink water often and avoid sodas and other drinks. Also remember to wash your face at the end of the day to clean the skin and do use a good moisturizer too..

I will be writing a short book soon about the effect of computer use induced dehydration on body functions. Please read that for more information on this subject when it comes out. Also read my online blogs on this important subject.

As this is a short book, this is all the information I will be providing in this short book

Chapter 5
How effective are Air Purifiers

There is a lot of talk around about air purifiers some people say they are good and beneficial to the health of asthma sufferers some others say they are bad.

The truth is that air purifiers are good if used correctly. The problem is that some people do not know that certain things have to be in place for air purifiers to provide the benefit they should.

One thing we all have to realize is that the whole of nature is coded which means things have to be in a certain way to operate effectively or else they will breakdown. A second thing we need to know is that introducing anything not a part of the code is like putting a virus in a computer system.

Consequently since air is supposed to be in a certain composition and certain things need to be in place to have that composition, the only way to have good quality air in the right configuration is to ensure all the components as far as we know are in place to at least a certain degree.

Hence as someone who had to use a filter before I started to get relief, this is what I learned from experience needs to be in place:

1. Sunlight filtering into the room where air is being filtered. The air outside needs sunlight to be balanced hence inside air needs some sunlight even if it is filtered in through glass windows or wooden shutters that have spaces in between the bars allowing enough sunlight in.

2. Natural outside air needs to be allowed in even if only through a crack i.e. crack open the window

3. The capacity of the air filter to produce negative ions must match the amount of artificial light in the room. If there is more artificial light producing all kinds of toxic light fields and chemicals beyond the capacity of the purifier to cope with it will not work well. It will be overwhelmed.

The more artificial light there is the higher the capacity of your air purifier needs to be and also the more outside air and sunlight you need to ensure the purifier works properly.

I have also discovered that it helps to have small indoor live plants such as the in the room. Do not put too many just one small one will do in a standard living room of 10' by 8'. They absorb some of the positive ions and produce negative ones. They also absorb some of the CO_2 i.e. carbon dioxide in the air.

Chapter 6
Nutrition and Exercises

In addition to the various solutions suggested in earlier chapters, there are also things one can do in terms of nutrition and exercise

Nutrition
It is important to realize that there is a limit to how much of artificial substance not coded to our being that our system can take before the soul level where the biochemicals that handle these issues become overwhelmed.

It is therefore important to reduce the amount of toxic substance we introduce to the system.

If we are already computer users, which automatically introduces a high level of toxins by way of artificial light and other chemicals our use exposes us to, it is important that we avoid the toxic chemicals, pesticides and herbicides inherent in conventional food.

Organic would be the way to go. Not that organic is perfect because most of the seeds of our food are no longer in the original way and have been tampered with and in addition a lot of our soils have already been damaged.

Hence even though they have been rehabilitated it will take a long, long time of correct cropping and use of the old way of fallowing which allows the land to rest every seven years or so over a long period of time to bring our soils back.

This will only work if the water supplies and other environmental issues are not damaged in some other way.

Consequently eat organic fruits and vegetables, eat only foods in the way they are supposed to be. Do not look for convenience. So for example eat only seeded grapes and oranges. That is they way they were created to be and the life is in the seed.

Eat only organic whole grains as bread, pasta and so on.

Apart from the common grains such as brown rice, whole wheat/wheat berries, there are old grains such as quinoa, millet, kashi and so on that have not been adulterated. Get them in health food stores and certain large supermarkets.

Take only milk from and eat only organic grass fed meat as cows, sheep and goat were only created to digest grass and that is all they can completely digest. They do not completely digest grains and the undigested part, which is toxic, is passed to us through the meat, milk and so on.

Hence though red meat with its high iron, amino acid and enzyme content is the best for us especially in the computer use environment that uses up a lot of all these nutrients, we have poisoned the natural safety measure provided by our creator to empower our body handle the stress.

Poultry does not have enough of these nutrients and consequently many people avoiding red meat are deficient in them. Meanwhile people eating conventional red meat are eating manmade toxins with their meat.

There is obviously a need for us to rethink our current food policies as we are killing ourselves by willfully destroying everything put in nature to keep us healthy in the greedy search for money at all cost.

This is nothing more than slow suicide.

Exercise
The best daily exercise is a long walk. Walk as much as you can. This is the way we were created to exercise our bodies.

Outdoors exercises of any sort are also very important and it does not have to be fore long. In my case I do 2 to 5 minutes outdoor exercises daily to complement my walking and indoor exercises. Remember to warm up before rigorous exercises and cool down afterwards i.e. do some warm up and cool down exercise.

You may consider joining an outdoor exercise early morning boot camp that do exercises that follow the body's natural exercise regimen.

I will be writing an exercise for computer users book in the future. Be sure to get it when it is published. Meanwhile do the best you can. There is a lot of exercise information available online and at gyms. Discuss them all with your doctor.

A warning. Do exercises that are exercises. Do not add anything else. Hence no yoga just exercises to avoid new issues.

Remember let the sunlight in when doing indoor exercises. There are many good exercises that help in working up the shoulder, neck, chest, back and abdominal muscles areas that are critical for lung and heart functions. Ask your doctor for advise before getting into any regimen.

The gym is also good and many have trainers on hand to provide assistance.

Exercise your eyes and brain by reading outside with the light of the sun daily. I have discovered that the best thing to read this way for maximum effect is the human machine user manual we call the Bible or Scriptures.

There are also certain outdoor eye exercises that help to exercise the eye muscles. I do some everyday and I also do some facial muscle and scalp exercises a few times a week

Detoxify

Detoxify using juice fasting with the assistance of your doctor who can monitor you and make changes to your fast if required.

Today we have a lot of soy in most things we eat however its estrogen is not well tolerated by our bodies which is why it is only eaten as condiment by Asians who introduced us to this grain. Therefore be careful.

Finally remember to pray. I would not be here and you would not be reading this book without that.

I will not be politically correct but will tell you what I have found works and which even medical science has abundant evidence of – Pray in the name of Jesus for that is what the manual instructs us to do. That is what is in the code and that is what will work.

Chapter 7
Summary and Conclusion

For a long time we have been looking at environmental induced allergy as being induced by pollutants in the air without acknowledging that environmental pollutants also emanate from artificial light.

Indeed anything that is not natural and consequently not part of the natural code of nature will be a pollutant to anything natural.

We all need to change the way we have been looking at the issue of the health effects of computer use if we want to remain a healthy prosperous population on earth.

One thing though, you must not self diagnose just look for a doctor who is ready to use other measures apart from medication as you will need close monitoring and some tests to identify what is depleted or missing in your body's system as a result of your computer use. These tests do not show everything but are a good starting point.

Computers are here to stay and can never be as safe as claimed. The computer use environment for example makes us look directly at a source of light to read, which is contrary to our natural way of never looking directly at the sun (our natural source of reading light).
Our problem is that we find it difficult to accept truth that makes us feel uncomfortable or need to look too closely at ourselves, or that imposes discipline, which we erroneously misinterpret as threatening our freedom instead of acknowledging it as preventing us from harming ourselves

We like to think we know everything and are in charge when in fact like every other machine we are under control. In fact no one has any thought of their own, we receive thoughts it is the one we accept and act upon that become ours and shape our lives.

There is also a consequence for every action as we are coded living machines and the consequence of every decision is part of our script.

Hence if we put in place measures that would allow us to use technology without self destroying, we will not self destroy but if we fail to change our ways then we will get hurt as a result of our willful ignorance.

Note To The Reader:

About the author:

Adetutu Ijose, is a technology and accounting professional with over 25 years of intensive computer use exposure who suffered life threatening computer related health conditions the doctors could neither diagnose not treat.

In desperation and with a good knowledge of codes and how they work she studied the human computer user manual we call the Bible until she was able to understand why and how the computer hurts our body's system as well as the preventative and repair kits placed in nature by our maker.

One of the issues she had was lung murmurs though she had no history of asthma or allergies. She also had lung congestion with a blocked nose and was sneezing all, which seemed to indicate she had somehow developed an allergy or asthma however normal allergy and cold medications did not help.

She began to realize that the issue was the computer use environment as she began to feel the heat of the light fields coming off the computer and the artificial lighting in the room where she worked. In addition the pollen that had never affected her before and the dust in the room became a factor making life unbearable.

A look at the user manual called the Bible revealed the problem. The air was imbalanced and the soul area and its biochemicals sere overwhelmed and were only presenting the discomfort in the best way available from the ways provided in the body's database (the manual tells us this database is located in the heart which passes the information to our brain and nerve network that then executes the necessary action).

After observing that many cashiers at supermarket working with computerized cash registers, friends who had computer use related work and others who asked her for help all had this issue as well as report in the news that asthma was on the rise for unknown reasons, she realized it was important for her to make the information she had public in a bid to help everyone.

She is now passing on her understanding about the contributory effect of computer use to the increasing asthma and allergy trends to everyone so others can receive help and avoid preventable devastating consequences of computer use.

Adetutu Ijose is a speaker on the subject of computer use induced health conditions. She is also a contributor to several online article websites and blogs including content sites associatedcontent.com and examiner.com. She has also been interviewed on radio.

To schedule a speaking or consulting engagement, interviews and so on with the author, please contact Adetutu Ijose at http://www.foodsthathealdaily.com.

For Adetutu Ijose's online press kit or for press releases and other media matters and inquiries, please go to http://lessosilearnedthehardway.com/AdetutuIjoseMedia PressKit.aspx

Discover other titles by Adetutu Ijose to help you better understand responsible computer use and how computer use affect us all as well as what we need to do to prevent

and manage these issues at
www.foodsthathealydaily.com, www.amazon.com and
other online stores. Ebook versions of this and other
books by Adetutu Ijose are available at amazon.com,
Barnes and Nobles, Smashword.com and other ebook
stores. A complete list is provided below.

Connect with Adetutu Ijose Online:
Facebook: http://www.facebook.com/home.php

Computer Use Induced Health Conditions related books by
Adetutu Ijose as at the time of writing are:

1. *Lessons I Learned the Hard Way: How to Identify,
    Minimize, Treat and Manage Computer Related
    Health Condition*

2. *Computer Related Health Condition: Understanding
    the Human Computer*

3. *Healing Juicing Smoothie and Milk Shake Recipes:
    Juices, Smoothies and Milk Shakes that Help the
    Body Achieve its Self Healing Process*

4. *Healing Meals Recipe: Meals that Help the Body
    Achieve its Self Healing Process*

5. *Cyber Bullying: How and Why Bullies operate*

6. *Global Epidemic: The Human Abuse of the
    Computer*

7. *Computer Use Addiction and Withdrawal Syndrome:
    What You Need to Know*

For other titles published after this book – *Allergies,
Asthma and Computer Use: The Contributory Effects of*

Computer Use to Allergies and Asthma Trends, please go to amazon.com and other online stores or visit my website www.foodsthathealdaily.com

Note to Doctors - Supplementation

It is very important to work with medical professionals.

Because of the various issues and depletion of nutrients that occur in computer use, it is important to get complete whole body chemistry analysis done analyzing the blood, urine and stool at the minimum to determine as much as possible what has been depleted in order to determine the best nutritional diet to embark upon and to determine if supplementation is necessary.

This analysis does not reveal everything but it is a very important starting point. It should be repeated as needed to track progress and determine necessary changes required in the treatment program.

When I became ill ing what was wrong. All I knew was that there was this asthma/ allergy like part of the problem that did not get better with conventional medicine.

I did not realize that it was the effect of light, chemical and other imbalances in the air.

If the patient is already badly hurt, I will recommend getting a homeopathic allergy remedy. Use only non-spray remedies to avoid worsening the situation. I used the one produced by BioAllers I used both the indoor and outdoor tablets. I also used a herbal tincture called lung tonic, and a ginger/garlic/apple cider vinegar/ Cayenne pepper mixture.

Please email me using the information provided in "Note to the Reader" if you need more details on how to use these remedies and all the other measures I took because of the severity of my issue and because it took a long time for me to understand what was going on,.

In addition, there could be a need for GABA and melatonin supplementation if stress and anxiety are manifested. Another thing that may be required there are behavioral issues is Rhodolia Rosea.

For computer use induced asthmas and allergy, there are other issues such as magnesium, zinc, iron, Vitamin D, B, C and other mineral and vitamin supplementation, but in order to ensure people go to their doctors, I will only go this far. I invite doctors to get in touch with me via the email address provided in "Note to the reader" for more information on supplementation. You can also read my book *Lessons I Learned the Hard way*.

Computer use induced health conditions should never be self diagnosed and treated without medical help to monitor the process. It is very dangerous to try to do it on your own. Get your doctor my books and get him or her to contact me for things like checklists, supplementation and other matters I consider too risky to provide to the general public.

References

1-1 2009 data for Centers for Disease and Prevention (CDC) r Asthma data for the US available at http://www.cdc.gov/nchs/fastats/asthma.htm

1-2 2006 data for Centers for Disease and Prevention (CDC) r Asthma data for the US available at - Summary Health Statistics for U.S. Children: National Health Interview Survey, 2006 http://www.cdc.gov/nchs/data/series/sr_10/sr10_234.pdf

1-3 2003-2005 Centers for Disease and Prevention (CDC) r Asthma data for the US available at http://www.cdc.gov/nchs/data/hestat/asthma03-05/asthma03-05.htm

1-4 1980-2005 and 1980-2005 Centers for Disease and Prevention (CDC) r Asthma data for the US available at

1980-2004 http://www.cdc.gov/mmwr/preview/mmwrhtml/ss5608a1.htm

1980-2005 http://www.cdc.gov/nchs/data/ad/ad381.pdf

1-2 CDC Health E –Stat Asthma Prevalence, Health Care Use and Mortality: United States, 2003-05 http://www.cdc.gov/nchs/data/hestat/asthma03-05/asthma03-05.htm

2-1 World Health Organization (WHO) Asthma Definition available at http://www.who.int/respiratory/asthma/definition/en/

2-2 Mayo clinics Allergy definition available at
http://www.mayoclinic.com/health/allergies/DS01118

2-3 The advanced data for vital and Health Statistics for
the CDC – Number 381 published in December 12 2006
revised December 29, 2006 - The State of Childhood
Asthma, United States, 1980–2005 by Lara J. Akinbami,
M.D., Office of Analysis and Epidemiology
http://www.cdc.gov/nchs/data/ad/ad381.pdf

2-4 CDC/National Health Interview Survey (NHIS) Data
2001 to 2009 data
 http://www.cdc.gov/asthma/nhis/default.htm

2-5 Article by Anisimov VN; Zabezhinski_ MA;
Muratov EI; Popovich IG; Arutiunian AV; Oparina TI;
Prokopenko VM on the effect of radiation from a
personal computer video terminal on estrus function,
melatonin level, and free radical processes in laboratory
rodents published in the journal *Biofi zika [Biofi zika]*
1998 Jan-Feb; Vol. 43 (1), pp. 165-70.

4-1 Paper presented by Dr. Neil Cherry associate
professor of environmental health, Lincoln University,
New Zealand on the effects of electromagnetic fields to
a group of European parliament MPs in 2000 available
in libraries and at http://beyondcreativity.blogs.com/fi
les/cherry-evidence-that-electromagnetic-radiation-is-
genotoxic-2002. pdf,
http://www.livingplanet.be/NeilCherry2002.pdf.

INDEX

A

Addition, 12, 14, 15, 18, 21, 28, 29, 33, 39
Air, 10, 18, 22, 23, 24, 25, 26, 27, 28, 29, 31, 32, 37, 39
Allergen, 10
Allergies, 5, 8, 10, 11, 12, 15, 16, 20, 24, 26, 39, 41, 44
Animal, 17
Antioxidant, 15
Artificial, 12, 14, 15, 16, 17, 18, 19, 23, 26, 27, 28, 32, 33, 37, 39
Asthma,5, 6, 8, 9, 10, 11, 12, 15, 16, 20, 24, 31, 39, 40, 41, 43, 44

B

Bacteria, 25
Balance, 13, 22, 23, 26
Bible, 5, 13, 16, 19, 36, 39
Biochemical, 15
Biochemicals, 13, 17, 18, 20, 22, 33, 39
Body, 12, 13, 15, 16, 18, 20, 22, 23, 28, 29, 30, 34, 35, 37, 39
Book, 3, 5, 6, 16, 21, 24, 26, 30, 35, 36, 41
Brown rice, 34

C

Cancer, 15, 23, 26
CDC, 8, 11, 43, 44
Cell Phones, 12
Chemicals, 12, 14, 16, 27, 32, 33
Chest congestion., 26
Children, 8, 9, 11
Claritin, 16

G

Goat, 34
Grapes, 34
Grass Fed, 34

H

Headaches, 5, 18, 23, 26
Hhealth, 5, 6, 8, 11, 16, 18, 24, 28, 31, 34, 37, 39, 40, 44
Heart Attack, 20
Herbicides, 27, 33
Hormone, 15
Human, 5, 16, 19, 36, 39
Humans, 13, 17, 22

I

Imbalance, 18, 22, 23, 27
Imbalance, 24
Imbalanced, 18, 28, 39
Immune, 10, 12
Indoors, 22
Ion, 24, 25
Ionization, 24
Ions, 17, 24, 34

K

Kashi, 34

L

Lessons, 16, 21, 26, 27, 41
Life, 5, 6, 11, 13, 14, 15, 16, 19, 20, 22, 34, 39
Lifeless, 14, 20, 27
Lifelessness, 20
Lifestyle, 6

P

Pesticides, 27, 33
Physical, 13, 14, 22, 25
Pigmentation, 22
Pollutants, 37
Poultry, 34
Pray, 36
Prayer, 5
Programmer, 17, 19
Purifiers, 31

Q

Quinoa, 34

R

Receptors, 12, 14, 28, 29
Red Meat, 34
Repair, 15, 20, 39
Research, 16
Resources, 14
Respiratory, 8, 11, 20, 43

S

Scientific, 11
Seasonal affective disorders, 26
Seeds, 33
Sensitivity, 10, 12, 14, 23, 26
Sensors, 14
Sheep, 34
Skin, 11, 23, 26, 28, 29, 30
Sneezing, 5, 15, 23, 39
Solutions, 33
Soul, 13, 14, 20, 33, 39
Spirit, 14, 20
Stimulates, 15, 17, 22